DIABETIC VEGAN COOKBOOKS FOR TYPE 2 DIABETES

30-Day Meal Plan & Delicious Vegan Recipes

T. John

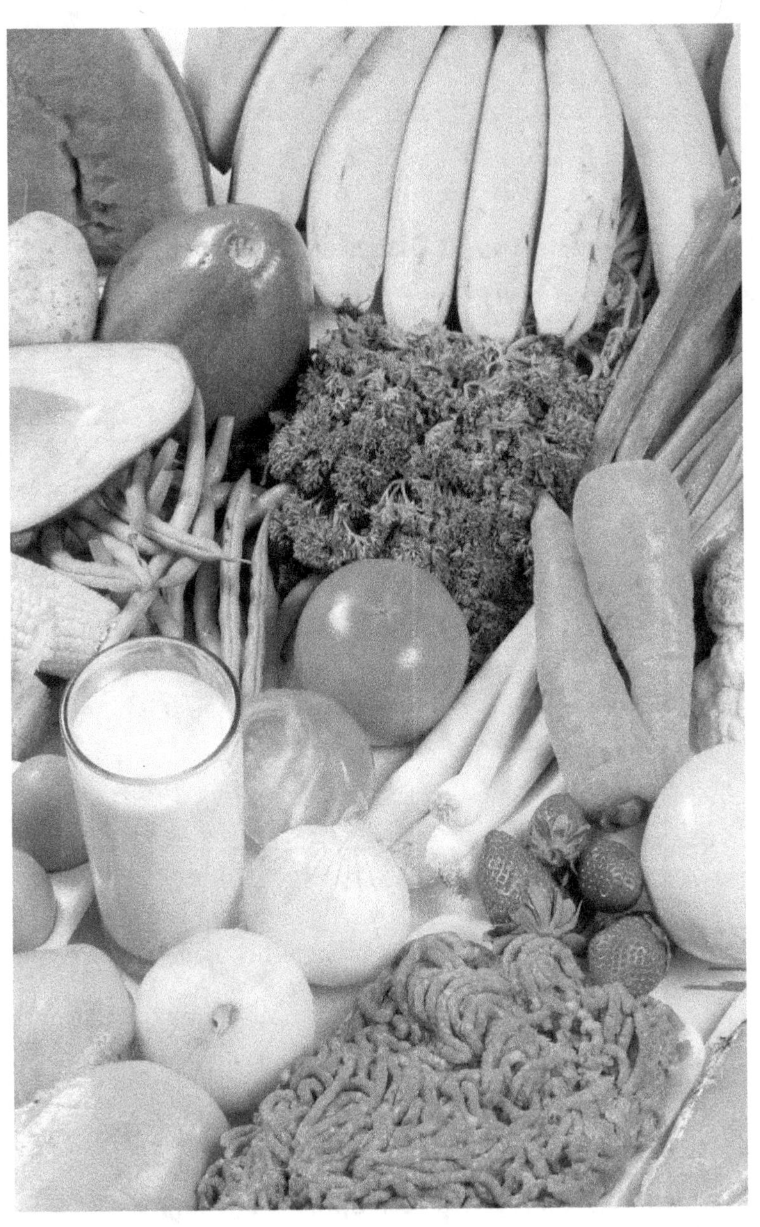

TABLE OF CONTENTS

Chapter 5: Snacks and Appetizers 84

CONCLUSION 141

INTRODUCTION

Type 2 diabetes, a chronic condition affecting millions worldwide, can feel overwhelming. But amidst the confusion, embracing a vegan lifestyle and setting realistic health goals can empower you to manage your condition and reclaim a sense of control.

Understanding Type 2 Diabetes:

Imagine your body as a bustling city, with insulin acting as the traffic cop, directing glucose (energy) from your bloodstream to your cells. In type 2 diabetes, this system malfunctions. Your cells become resistant to insulin, leading to high blood sugar levels.

Veganism: A Powerhouse for Managing Diabetes:

A vegan diet, rich in fruits, vegetables, legumes, whole grains, and nuts, can be a powerful tool in your diabetes management arsenal. Here's why:

1. Lowers blood sugar: Plant-based foods are naturally low in fat and processed sugars, helping you regulate blood sugar levels.

2. Promotes weight management: Maintaining a healthy weight is crucial for managing diabetes. Vegan diets tend to be lower in calories and promote satiety, aiding weight loss or maintenance.

3. Improves heart health: Type 2 diabetes increases your risk of heart disease. Vegan diets, rich in fruits and vegetables, can lower your cholesterol and blood pressure, protecting your heart.

4. Boosts gut health: A healthy gut microbiome is essential for overall health, including managing diabetes. Plant-based foods are rich in prebiotics, which nourish gut bacteria, aiding in glucose control.

Setting Realistic Health Goals:

While adopting a vegan lifestyle can work wonders, it's crucial to set realistic goals to sustain long-term success. Here are some tips:

1. Start small: Don't try to overhaul your diet overnight. Begin by incorporating more plant-based meals into your week gradually.

2. Focus on progress, not perfection: Slips are inevitable. Don't get discouraged; pick yourself up and recommit to your goals.

3. Seek support: Join online communities, connect with fellow vegans, or consult a nutritionist for guidance and encouragement.

4. Celebrate your wins: Acknowledge your achievements, no matter how small. This keeps you motivated and reinforces your positive choices.

Embracing a vegan lifestyle isn't just about dietary changes; it's about a holistic approach to health and well-being. By understanding type 2 diabetes, harnessing the power of a plant-based diet, and setting realistic goals, you can empower yourself to manage your condition and pave the way for a healthier, happier life.

Remember, your journey is unique. Embrace your individuality, listen to your body, and make choices that resonate with you. With the right mindset and support, you can thrive despite your diagnosis and write a new chapter of health and empowerment in your life.

Chapter 1: 30-Day Meal Plan

Week 1:

Day 1:

- Breakfast: Quinoa and Berry Breakfast Bowl
- Lunch: Lentil and Vegetable Soup
- Dinner: Eggplant and Spinach Lasagna
- Snacks: Guacamole with Veggie Sticks
- Dessert: Berry and Almond Tart

Day 2:

- Breakfast: Avocado and Tomato Toast
- Lunch: Quinoa and Black Bean Salad
- Dinner: Chickpea and Vegetable Stir-Fry
- Snacks: Roasted Red Pepper Hummus
- Dessert: Vegan Chocolate Avocado Mousse

Day 3:

- Breakfast: Chia Seed Pudding with Almond Milk
- Lunch: Grilled Portobello Mushroom Wraps
- Dinner: Stuffed Acorn Squash with Quinoa

- Snacks: Vegan Spinach and Artichoke Dip
- Dessert: Pumpkin Pie with Oat Crust

Day 4:

- Breakfast: Spinach and Mushroom Vegan Omelette
- Lunch: Cauliflower and Chickpea Curry
- Dinner: Vegan Chili with Kidney Beans
- Snacks: Edamame and Sesame Seed Crackers
- Dessert: Coconut and Lime Sorbet

Day 5:

- Breakfast: Overnight Oats with Fresh Fruits
- Lunch: Sweet Potato and Kale Buddha Bowl
- Dinner: Cauliflower and Potato Curry
- Snacks: Spicy Avocado Salsa
- Dessert: Apple Cinnamon Baked Oatmeal

Day 6:

- Breakfast: Sweet Potato and Black Bean Breakfast Burrito
- Lunch: Mediterranean Stuffed Bell Peppers
- Dinner: Zoodle (Zucchini Noodle) Alfredo

- Snacks: Baked Sweet Potato Fries
- Dessert: Chocolate Chip Banana Bread

Day 7:

- Breakfast: Vegan Pancakes with Sugar-Free Syrup
- Lunch: Spaghetti Squash Primavera
- Dinner: Mexican Quinoa Casserole
- Snacks: Stuffed Grape Leaves with Tofu
- Dessert: Vegan Lemon Bars

Week 2:

Day 8:

- Breakfast: Tofu Scramble with Vegetables
- Lunch: Vegan Tacos with Walnut "Meat"
- Dinner: Portobello Mushroom Steaks
- Snacks: Vegan Caprese Skewers
- Dessert: Raspberry Chia Seed Pudding

Day 9:

- Breakfast: Banana Walnut Muffins
- Lunch: Cucumber and Avocado Sushi Rolls
- Dinner: Ratatouille with Herbed Polenta

- Snacks: Kale Chips with Nutritional Yeast
- Dessert: Almond Butter and Jelly Thumbprint Cookies

Day 10:

- Breakfast: Berry and Almond Smoothie Bowl
- Lunch: Roasted Red Pepper and Hummus Wrap
- Dinner: Thai Basil Tofu Stir-Fry
- Snacks: Buffalo Cauliflower Bites
- Dessert: Dark Chocolate Covered Strawberries

Day 11:

- Breakfast: Chickpea Flour Crepes with Spinach
- Lunch: Broccoli and Almond Stir-Fry
- Dinner: Wild Rice and Vegetable Pilaf
- Snacks: Vegan Cheese and Crackers
- Dessert: Blueberry and Lemon Coconut Bliss Balls

Day 12:

- Breakfast: Mediterranean Quinoa Salad
- Lunch: Black-Eyed Pea and Vegetable Stew
- Dinner: Spiced Lentil and Vegetable Skewers

- Snacks: Avocado and Black Bean Salsa

- Dessert: Pistachio and Cranberry Biscotti

Day 13:

- Breakfast: Green Smoothie with Kale and Pineapple

- Lunch: Vegan Caesar Salad with Crispy Chickpeas

- Dinner: Creamy Mushroom and Spinach Risotto

- Snacks: Almond and Cranberry Energy Bites

- Dessert: Mango and Coconut Rice Pudding

Day 14:

- Breakfast: Zucchini and Carrot Muffins

- Lunch: Thai-Inspired Coconut Soup

- Dinner: Vegan Jambalaya with Okra

- Snacks: Cucumber Rolls with Vegan Cream Cheese

- Dessert: Chocolate Peanut Butter Cupcakes

Week 3:

Day 15:

- Breakfast: Peanut Butter and Banana Toast

- Lunch: BBQ Tempeh and Slaw Sandwich

- Dinner: Butternut Squash and Sage Risotto

- Snacks: Roasted Chickpeas with Smoky Paprika
- Dessert: Avocado Chocolate Mousse Tart

Day 16:

- Breakfast: Quinoa and Berry Breakfast Bowl
- Lunch: Lentil and Vegetable Soup
- Dinner: Eggplant and Spinach Lasagna
- Snacks: Guacamole with Veggie Sticks
- Dessert: Berry and Almond Tart

Day 17:

- Breakfast: Avocado and Tomato Toast
- Lunch: Quinoa and Black Bean Salad
- Dinner: Chickpea and Vegetable Stir-Fry
- Snacks: Roasted Red Pepper Hummus
- Dessert: Vegan Chocolate Avocado Mousse

Day 18:

- Breakfast: Chia Seed Pudding with Almond Milk
- Lunch: Grilled Portobello Mushroom Wraps
- Dinner: Stuffed Acorn Squash with Quinoa
- Snacks: Vegan Spinach and Artichoke Dip

- Dessert: Pumpkin Pie with Oat Crust

Day 19:

- Breakfast: Spinach and Mushroom Vegan Omelette
- Lunch: Cauliflower and Chickpea Curry
- Dinner: Vegan Chili with Kidney Beans
- Snacks: Edamame and Sesame Seed Crackers
- Dessert: Coconut and Lime Sorbet

Day 20:

- Breakfast: Overnight Oats with Fresh Fruits
- Lunch: Sweet Potato and Kale Buddha Bowl
- Dinner: Cauliflower and Potato Curry
- Snacks: Spicy Avocado Salsa
- Dessert: Apple Cinnamon Baked Oatmeal

Day 21:

- Breakfast: Sweet Potato and Black Bean Breakfast Burrito
- Lunch: Mediterranean Stuffed Bell Peppers
- Dinner: Zoodle (Zucchini Noodle) Alfredo
- Snacks: Baked Sweet Potato Fries

- Dessert: Chocolate Chip Banana Bread

Week 4:

Day 22:

- Breakfast: Vegan Pancakes with Sugar-Free Syrup
- Lunch: Spaghetti Squash Primavera
- Dinner: Mexican Quinoa Casserole
- Snacks: Stuffed Grape Leaves with Tofu
- Dessert: Vegan Lemon Bars

Day 23:

- Breakfast: Tofu Scramble with Vegetables
- Lunch: Vegan Tacos with Walnut "Meat"
- Dinner: Portobello Mushroom Steaks
- Snacks: Vegan Caprese Skewers
- Dessert: Raspberry Chia Seed Pudding

Day 24:

- Breakfast: Banana Walnut Muffins
- Lunch: Cucumber and Avocado Sushi Rolls
- Dinner: Ratatouille with Herbed Polenta
- Snacks: Kale Chips with Nutritional Yeast

- Dessert: Almond Butter and Jelly Thumbprint Cookies

Day 25:

- Breakfast: Berry and Almond Smoothie Bowl
- Lunch: Roasted Red Pepper and Hummus Wrap
- Dinner: Thai Basil Tofu Stir-Fry
- Snacks: Buffalo Cauliflower Bites
- Dessert: Dark Chocolate Covered Strawberries

Day 26:

- Breakfast: Chickpea Flour Crepes with Spinach
- Lunch: Broccoli and Almond Stir-Fry
- Dinner: Wild Rice and Vegetable Pilaf
- Snacks: Vegan Cheese and Crackers
- Dessert: Blueberry and Lemon Coconut Bliss Balls

Day 27:

- Breakfast: Mediterranean Quinoa Salad
- Lunch: Black-Eyed Pea and Vegetable Stew
- Dinner: Spiced Lentil and Vegetable Skewers
- Snacks: Avocado and Black Bean Salsa

- Dessert: Pistachio and Cranberry Biscotti

Day 28:

- Breakfast: Green Smoothie with Kale and Pineapple
- Lunch: Vegan Caesar Salad with Crispy Chickpeas
- Dinner: Creamy Mushroom and Spinach Risotto
- Snacks: Almond and Cranberry Energy Bites
- Dessert: Mango and Coconut Rice Pudding

Day 29:

- Breakfast: Zucchini and Carrot Muffins
- Lunch: Thai-Inspired Coconut Soup
- Dinner: Vegan Jambalaya with Okra
- Snacks: Cucumber Rolls with Vegan Cream Cheese
- Dessert: Chocolate Peanut Butter Cupcakes

Day 30:

- Breakfast: Peanut Butter and Banana Toast
- Lunch: BBQ Tempeh and Slaw Sandwich
- Dinner: Butternut Squash and Sage Risotto
- Snacks: Roasted Chickpeas with Smoky Paprika
- Dessert: Avocado Chocolate Mousse Tart

Chapter 2: Breakfast Recipes

These recipes are thoughtfully crafted to provide both flavor and nutrition, setting the perfect tone for your day. Whether you're a seasoned breakfast enthusiast or just starting your journey, these recipes offer a diverse array of delicious options to keep your mornings both exciting and health-conscious.

Quinoa and Berry Breakfast Bowl

Ingredients:

- 1/2 cup cooked quinoa
- 1 cup mixed berries (strawberries, blueberries, raspberries)
- 1 tablespoon chia seeds
- 1 tablespoon almond butter
- 1 teaspoon honey (optional)

Instructions:

1. In a bowl, layer cooked quinoa.

2. Top with mixed berries, chia seeds, and almond
    butter.

3. Drizzle with honey for added sweetness if desired.

Nutrition Information (per serving):

- Calories: 300

- Protein: 8g

- Carbohydrates: 45g

- Fat: 10g

- Fiber: 9g

- Sugar: 10g

- Portion Size: 1 serving

Avocado and Tomato Toast

Ingredients:

- 1 slice whole-grain bread

- 1/2 ripe avocado, mashed

- 1/2 cup cherry tomatoes, halved

- Sprinkle of salt and pepper

- Optional: red pepper flakes for heat

Instructions:

1. Toast the whole-grain bread to your liking.

2. Spread mashed avocado evenly on the toast.

3. Top with halved cherry tomatoes.

4. Sprinkle with salt, pepper, and optional red pepper flakes.

Nutrition Information (per serving):

- Calories: 220
- Protein: 5g
- Carbohydrates: 20g
- Fat: 14g
- Fiber: 7g
- Sugar: 2g
- Portion Size: 1 serving

Chia Seed Pudding with Almond Milk

Ingredients:

- 2 tablespoons chia seeds
- 1/2 cup unsweetened almond milk
- 1/2 teaspoon vanilla extract
- Fresh berries for topping

Instructions:

1. Mix chia seeds, almond milk, and vanilla extract in a jar.
2. Refrigerate for at least 2 hours or overnight.
3. Stir well before serving and top with fresh berries.

Nutrition Information (per serving):

- Calories: 150
- Protein: 4g
- Carbohydrates: 15g
- Fat: 8g
- Fiber: 10g
- Sugar: 2g
- Portion Size: 1 serving

Spinach and Mushroom Vegan Omelette

Ingredients:

- 1 cup spinach, chopped
- 1/2 cup mushrooms, sliced
- 1/4 cup red bell pepper, diced

- 1/2 cup firm tofu, crumbled

- 1 tablespoon nutritional yeast

- Salt and pepper to taste

Instructions:

1. Sauté spinach, mushrooms, and red bell pepper in a pan.

2. Add crumbled tofu and nutritional yeast.

3. Season with salt and pepper, cook until heated through.

Nutrition Information (per serving):

- Calories: 180

- Protein: 12g

- Carbohydrates: 8g

- Fat: 12g

- Fiber: 4g

- Sugar: 2g

- Portion Size: 1 serving

Overnight Oats with Fresh Fruits

Ingredients:

- 1/2 cup rolled oats
- 1/2 cup unsweetened almond milk
- 1/2 banana, sliced
- Handful of berries (strawberries, blueberries)
- 1 tablespoon almond butter

Instructions:

1. In a jar, combine rolled oats and almond milk.
2. Layer with sliced banana and berries.
3. Refrigerate overnight.
4. Before serving, top with almond butter.

Nutrition Information (per serving):

- Calories: 280
- Protein: 8g
- Carbohydrates: 38g
- Fat: 12g
- Fiber: 7g
- Sugar: 10g
- Portion Size: 1 serving

Sweet Potato and Black Bean Breakfast Burrito

Ingredients:

- 1 whole-grain tortilla
- 1/2 cup sweet potato, cooked and mashed
- 1/4 cup black beans, drained and rinsed
- Salsa and guacamole for topping

Instructions:

1. Spread sweet potato on the tortilla.
2. Add black beans and top with salsa and guacamole.
3. Roll into a burrito and enjoy.

Nutrition Information (per serving):

- Calories: 320
- Protein: 10g
- Carbohydrates: 55g
- Fat: 8g
- Fiber: 12g
- Sugar: 5g
- Portion Size: 1 serving

Vegan Pancakes with Sugar-Free Syrup

Ingredients:

- 1 cup whole wheat flour
- 1 tablespoon baking powder
- 1 tablespoon flaxseed meal mixed with 3 tablespoons water (flax egg)
- 1 cup almond milk
- 1 tablespoon maple syrup
- Sugar-free syrup for topping

Instructions:

1. In a bowl, mix flour and baking powder.
2. Add flax egg, almond milk, and maple syrup. Mix well.
3. Cook pancakes on a griddle.
4. Top with sugar-free syrup.

Nutrition Information (per serving):

- Calories: 230
- Protein: 7g
- Carbohydrates: 45g

- Fat: 3g

- Fiber: 7g

- Sugar: 5g

- Portion Size: 1 serving

Tofu Scramble with Vegetables

Ingredients:

- 1/2 block firm tofu, crumbled

- 1 cup mixed vegetables (bell peppers, onions, tomatoes)

- 1 teaspoon turmeric

- Salt and pepper to taste

Instructions:

1. Sauté mixed vegetables until tender.

2. Add crumbled tofu and turmeric.

3. Season with salt and pepper, cook until heated through.

Nutrition Information (per serving):

- Calories: 210

- Protein: 15g

- Carbohydrates: 12g

- Fat: 12g

- Fiber: 5g

- Sugar: 4g

- Portion Size: 1 serving

Banana Walnut Muffins

Ingredients:

- 1 cup whole wheat flour

- 1/2 cup mashed ripe bananas

- 1/4 cup maple syrup

- 1/4 cup chopped walnuts

- 1/4 cup almond milk

- 1 teaspoon baking powder

Instructions:

1. Preheat oven to 350°F (175°C).

2. In a bowl, mix flour and baking powder.

3. In a separate bowl, combine mashed bananas, maple syrup, and almond milk.

4. Add wet ingredients to dry, fold in chopped walnuts.

5. Spoon batter into muffin cups and bake for 20-25 minutes.

Nutrition Information (per serving):

- Calories: 180
- Protein: 5g
- Carbohydrates: 30g
- Fat: 5g
- Fiber: 4g
- Sugar: 12g
- Portion Size: 1 muffin

Berry and Almond Smoothie Bowl

Ingredients:

- 1 cup mixed berries (strawberries, blueberries, raspberries)
- 1/2 banana, frozen
- 1/2 cup spinach leaves
- 1 tablespoon almond butter
- 1 cup almond milk
- Toppings: sliced almonds, chia seeds, shredded coconut

Instructions:

1. Blend berries, banana, spinach, almond butter, and almond milk until smooth.
2. Pour into a bowl and add desired toppings.

Nutrition Information (per serving):

- Calories: 250
- Protein: 8g
- Carbohydrates: 35g
- Fat: 11g
- Fiber: 10g
- Sugar: 15g
- Portion Size: 1 serving

Chickpea Flour Crepes with Spinach

Ingredients:

- 1 cup chickpea flour
- 1 1/4 cups water
- 1 cup fresh spinach, chopped
- 1/2 cup cherry tomatoes, sliced
- 1/4 cup red onion, finely chopped
- 1 tablespoon olive oil

Instructions:

1. Whisk chickpea flour and water until smooth.

2. Stir in chopped spinach, cherry tomatoes, and red onion.

3. Heat olive oil in a pan, pour batter to make crepes.

4. Cook until edges lift, then flip and cook the other side.

Nutrition Information (per serving):

- Calories: 220
- Protein: 10g
- Carbohydrates: 25g
- Fat: 10g
- Fiber: 6g
- Sugar: 4g
- Portion Size: 2 crepes

Mediterranean Quinoa Salad

Ingredients:

- 1 cup cooked quinoa
- 1/2 cup cucumber, diced
- 1/2 cup cherry tomatoes, halved

- 1/4 cup Kalamata olives, sliced
- 2 tablespoons red onion, finely chopped
- 2 tablespoons olive oil
- 1 tablespoon lemon juice

Instructions:

1. In a bowl, combine quinoa, cucumber, cherry tomatoes, olives, and red onion.
2. Drizzle with olive oil and lemon juice, toss to combine.

Nutrition Information (per serving):

- Calories: 280
- Protein: 7g
- Carbohydrates: 30g
- Fat: 15g
- Fiber: 5g
- Sugar: 2g
- Portion Size: 1 serving

Green Smoothie with Kale and Pineapple

Ingredients:

- 1 cup kale, stems removed
- 1/2 cup pineapple chunks
- 1/2 banana
- 1/2 cup coconut water
- 1 tablespoon chia seeds

Instructions:

1. Blend kale, pineapple, banana, and coconut water until smooth.
2. Add chia seeds and blend for a few more seconds.

Nutrition Information (per serving):

- Calories: 200
- Protein: 5g
- Carbohydrates: 40g
- Fat: 4g
- Fiber: 10g
- Sugar: 20g
- Portion Size: 1 serving

Zucchini and Carrot Muffins

Ingredients:

- 1 cup grated zucchini
- 1/2 cup grated carrot
- 1 cup whole wheat flour
- 1/2 cup maple syrup
- 1/4 cup coconut oil, melted
- 1 teaspoon baking powder

Instructions:

1. Preheat oven to 350°F (175°C).
2. In a bowl, mix grated zucchini, carrot, flour, maple syrup, coconut oil, and baking powder.
3. Spoon batter into muffin cups and bake for 20-25 minutes.

Nutrition Information (per serving):

- Calories: 180
- Protein: 4g
- Carbohydrates: 30g
- Fat: 6g
- Fiber: 4g

- Sugar: 15g

- Portion Size: 1 muffin

Peanut Butter and Banana Toast

Ingredients:

- 1 slice whole-grain bread

- 2 tablespoons peanut butter

- 1/2 banana, sliced

- Drizzle of honey (optional)

Instructions:

1. Toast the whole-grain bread to your liking.

2. Spread peanut butter on the toast.

3. Top with sliced banana.

4. Drizzle with honey for added sweetness if desired.

Nutrition Information (per serving):

- Calories: 280

- Protein: 8g

- Carbohydrates: 35g

- Fat: 13g

- Fiber: 6g

- Sugar: 14g

- Portion Size: 1 serving

Chapter 3: Lunch Recipes

Embark on a culinary journey that fuses flavors and nourishes your well-being with our collection of vibrant and delectable lunch recipes. From hearty soups to satisfying wraps, each dish is crafted to not only delight your taste buds but also align with a diabetic vegan lifestyle.

Lentil and Vegetable Soup

Ingredients:

- 1 cup green lentils, rinsed
- 1 onion, diced
- 2 carrots, sliced
- 2 celery stalks, chopped
- 3 cloves garlic, minced
- 1 can diced tomatoes
- 6 cups vegetable broth
- 1 teaspoon cumin
- 1 teaspoon paprika
- Salt and pepper to taste

Instructions:

1. In a large pot, sauté onions and garlic until fragrant.
2. Add lentils, carrots, celery, tomatoes, and vegetable broth.
3. Season with cumin, paprika, salt, and pepper.
4. Bring to a boil, then simmer until lentils are tender.
5. Serve hot.

Nutrition Information:

- Calories: 250
- Protein: 15g
- Carbohydrates: 45g
- Fat: 2g
- Fiber: 12g
- Sugar: 6g
- Portion Size: 1.5 cups

Quinoa and Black Bean Salad

Ingredients:

- 1 cup cooked quinoa
- 1 can black beans, drained and rinsed
- 1 bell pepper, diced

- 1 cup cherry tomatoes, halved

- 1/4 cup red onion, finely chopped

- 1/4 cup fresh cilantro, chopped

- 2 tablespoons olive oil

- 1 lime, juiced

- Salt and pepper to taste

Instructions:

1. In a large bowl, combine quinoa, black beans, bell pepper, tomatoes, red onion, and cilantro.

2. In a small bowl, whisk together olive oil, lime juice, salt, and pepper.

3. Pour the dressing over the salad and toss gently.

4. Chill in the refrigerator before serving.

Nutrition Information:

- Calories: 280

- Protein: 10g

- Carbohydrates: 40g

- Fat: 8g

- Fiber: 8g

- Sugar: 2g

- Portion Size: 1 cup

Grilled Portobello Mushroom Wraps

Ingredients:

- 4 large portobello mushrooms, cleaned and sliced
- 1 red onion, thinly sliced
- 1 bell pepper, thinly sliced
- 2 tablespoons balsamic vinegar
- 2 tablespoons olive oil
- 4 whole-grain tortillas
- Fresh spinach leaves
- Salt and pepper to taste

Instructions:

1. Marinate mushrooms, onions, and bell peppers in balsamic vinegar and olive oil.
2. Grill the vegetables until tender.
3. Warm tortillas and assemble with grilled veggies and fresh spinach.
4. Season with salt and pepper.
5. Roll into wraps and serve.

Nutrition Information:

- Calories: 220
- Protein: 6g
- Carbohydrates: 30g
- Fat: 10g
- Fiber: 6g
- Sugar: 5g
- Portion Size: 1 wrap

Cauliflower and Chickpea Curry

Ingredients:

- 1 cauliflower, cut into florets
- 1 can chickpeas, drained and rinsed
- 1 onion, finely chopped
- 3 cloves garlic, minced
- 1 tablespoon ginger, grated
- 1 can coconut milk
- 2 tablespoons curry powder
- 1 teaspoon turmeric
- Salt and pepper to taste
- Fresh cilantro for garnish

Instructions:

1. Sauté onions, garlic, and ginger until softened.
2. Add cauliflower, chickpeas, coconut milk, curry powder, and turmeric.
3. Simmer until cauliflower is tender.
4. Season with salt and pepper.
5. Garnish with fresh cilantro before serving.

Nutrition Information:

- Calories: 280
- Protein: 8g
- Carbohydrates: 25g
- Fat: 18g
- Fiber: 7g
- Sugar: 5g
- Portion Size: 1.5 cups

Sweet Potato and Kale Buddha Bowl

Ingredients:

- 2 sweet potatoes, cubed
- 2 cups kale, chopped
- 1 can chickpeas, roasted

- 1 avocado, sliced

- 2 tablespoons tahini

- 1 tablespoon lemon juice

- 1 tablespoon olive oil

- Salt and pepper to taste

Instructions:

1. Roast sweet potatoes and chickpeas until golden.

2. Massage kale with olive oil until wilted.

3. Assemble bowl with sweet potatoes, chickpeas, kale, and avocado.

4. Drizzle with tahini and lemon juice.

5. Season with salt and pepper.

Nutrition Information:

- Calories: 320

- Protein: 10g

- Carbohydrates: 45g

- Fat: 15g

- Fiber: 12g

- Sugar: 6g

- Portion Size: 2 cups

Mediterranean Stuffed Bell Peppers

Ingredients:

- 4 bell peppers, halved
- 1 cup quinoa, cooked
- 1 can chickpeas, mashed
- 1 cup cherry tomatoes, diced
- 1/2 cup Kalamata olives, chopped
- 1/4 cup red onion, finely chopped
- 2 tablespoons olive oil
- 1 tablespoon balsamic vinegar
- Fresh parsley for garnish

Instructions:

1. Preheat oven to 375°F (190°C).
2. In a bowl, mix quinoa, mashed chickpeas, tomatoes, olives, and red onion.
3. Stuff bell peppers with the mixture.
4. Drizzle with olive oil and balsamic vinegar.
5. Bake until peppers are tender.
6. Garnish with fresh parsley.

Nutrition Information:

- Calories: 240
- Protein: 8g
- Carbohydrates: 35g
- Fat: 8g
- Fiber: 9g
- Sugar: 6g
- Portion Size: 2 pepper halves

Spaghetti Squash Primavera

Ingredients:

- 1 spaghetti squash, halved
- 1 zucchini, julienned
- 1 carrot, julienned
- 1 bell pepper, thinly sliced
- 2 cloves garlic, minced
- 1 cup cherry tomatoes, halved
- 2 tablespoons olive oil
- 1 teaspoon Italian seasoning
- Salt and pepper to taste

Instructions:

1. Roast spaghetti squash in the oven.
2. In a pan, sauté zucchini, carrot, bell pepper, and garlic in olive oil.
3. Add cherry tomatoes and cook until softened.
4. Scrape spaghetti squash into strands and toss with vegetables.
5. Season with Italian seasoning, salt, and pepper.

Nutrition Information:

*   Calories: 220
*   Protein: 4g
*   Carbohydrates: 30g
*   Fat: 10g
*   Fiber: 8g
*   Sugar: 8g
*   Portion Size: 1.5 cups

Vegan Tacos with Walnut "Meat"

Ingredients:

*   1 cup walnuts, soaked
*   1 cup mushrooms, chopped

- 1 tablespoon soy sauce

- 1 teaspoon cumin

- 1 teaspoon chili powder

- 1/2 teaspoon paprika

- Corn tortillas

- Toppings: shredded lettuce, diced tomatoes, guacamole

Instructions:

1. Blend soaked walnuts, mushrooms, soy sauce, cumin, chili powder, and paprika until crumbly.
2. Heat walnut "meat" in a pan until browned.
3. Fill corn tortillas with walnut "meat" and desired toppings.

Nutrition Information:

- Calories: 180

- Protein: 6g

- Carbohydrates: 15g

- Fat: 12g

- Fiber: 5g

- Sugar: 2g

- Portion Size: 2 tacos

Cucumber and Avocado Sushi Rolls

Ingredients:

- 2 cups sushi rice, cooked
- 4 nori sheets
- 1 cucumber, julienned
- 1 avocado, sliced
- Soy sauce for dipping
- Pickled ginger and wasabi for serving

Instructions:

1. Place a nori sheet on a bamboo sushi mat.
2. Spread a thin layer of sushi rice over the nori.
3. Arrange cucumber and avocado along one edge.
4. Roll tightly, wetting the edge to seal.
5. Slice into sushi rolls and serve with soy sauce, pickled ginger, and wasabi.

Nutrition Information:

- Calories: 240
- Protein: 4g

- Carbohydrates: 45g

- Fat: 6g

- Fiber: 8g

- Sugar: 2g

- Portion Size: 6 pieces

Roasted Red Pepper and Hummus Wrap

Ingredients:

- 1 whole-grain wrap

- 1/2 cup hummus

- 1 roasted red pepper, sliced

- 1 cup mixed greens

- 1/4 cup cucumber, sliced

- 1 tablespoon balsamic glaze

Instructions:

1. Spread hummus over the whole-grain wrap.

2. Layer with roasted red pepper, mixed greens, and cucumber.

3. Drizzle with balsamic glaze.

4. Roll into a wrap and slice in half.

Nutrition Information:

- Calories: 300
- Protein: 8g
- Carbohydrates: 40g
- Fat: 12g
- Fiber: 10g
- Sugar: 5g
- Portion Size: 1 wrap

Broccoli and Almond Stir-Fry

Ingredients:

- 2 cups broccoli florets
- 1 bell pepper, sliced
- 1 carrot, julienned
- 1 cup snow peas
- 1/4 cup almonds, sliced
- 2 tablespoons soy sauce
- 1 tablespoon sesame oil
- 1 teaspoon ginger, grated
- 2 cloves garlic, minced

Instructions:

1. In a wok, stir-fry broccoli, bell pepper, carrot, and snow peas in sesame oil.
2. Add soy sauce, ginger, and garlic.
3. Continue to stir-fry until vegetables are tender.
4. Garnish with sliced almonds before serving.

Nutrition Information:

- Calories: 230
- Protein: 10g
- Carbohydrates: 25g
- Fat: 12g
- Fiber: 8g
- Sugar: 6g
- Portion Size: 1.5 cups

Black-Eyed Pea and Vegetable Stew

Ingredients:

- 1 cup dried black-eyed peas, soaked
- 1 onion, diced
- 2 carrots, sliced
- 2 celery stalks, chopped

- 1 bell pepper, diced

- 3 cloves garlic, minced

- 1 can diced tomatoes

- 6 cups vegetable broth

- 1 teaspoon thyme

- 1 bay leaf

- Salt and pepper to taste

Instructions:

1. Sauté onions, garlic, and celery until softened.
2. Add black-eyed peas, carrots, bell pepper, tomatoes, and vegetable broth.
3. Season with thyme, bay leaf, salt, and pepper.
4. Simmer until black-eyed peas are tender.
5. Remove bay leaf before serving.

Nutrition Information:

- Calories: 260

- Protein: 12g

- Carbohydrates: 45g

- Fat: 2g

- Fiber: 10g

- Sugar: 6g
- Portion Size: 1.5 cups

Vegan Caesar Salad with Crispy Chickpeas

Ingredients:

- 1 head romaine lettuce, chopped
- 1 cup cherry tomatoes, halved
- 1/4 cup vegan Caesar dressing
- 1/2 cup croutons
- 1/2 cup crispy chickpeas
- 2 tablespoons nutritional yeast
- Lemon wedges for serving

Instructions:

1. In a large bowl, toss romaine lettuce and cherry tomatoes.
2. Drizzle with vegan Caesar dressing and toss.
3. Top with croutons and crispy chickpeas.
4. Sprinkle with nutritional yeast.
5. Serve with lemon wedges.

Nutrition Information:

- Calories: 180
- Protein: 6g
- Carbohydrates: 25g
- Fat: 8g
- Fiber: 6g
- Sugar: 5g
- Portion Size: 2 cups

Thai-Inspired Coconut Soup

Ingredients:

- 1 tablespoon coconut oil
- 1 onion, diced
- 2 tablespoons red curry paste
- 1 can coconut milk
- 4 cups vegetable broth
- 1 cup shiitake mushrooms, sliced
- 1 cup bok choy, chopped
- 1 tablespoon soy sauce
- 1 tablespoon lime juice
- Fresh cilantro for garnish

Instructions:

1. In a pot, sauté onions in coconut oil.
2. Add red curry paste and stir.
3. Pour in coconut milk and vegetable broth.
4. Add mushrooms and bok choy.
5. Season with soy sauce and lime juice.
6. Simmer until vegetables are tender.
7. Garnish with fresh cilantro.

Nutrition Information:

- Calories: 240
- Protein: 6g
- Carbohydrates: 15g
- Fat: 20g
- Fiber: 4g
- Sugar: 5g
- Portion Size: 2 cups

BBQ Tempeh and Slaw Sandwich

Ingredients:

- 1 block tempeh, sliced
- 1/2 cup BBQ sauce

- 4 whole-grain buns
- 1 cup cabbage, shredded
- 1 carrot, grated
- 1/4 cup vegan mayonnaise
- 1 tablespoon apple cider vinegar
- Salt and pepper to taste

Instructions:

1. Marinate tempeh slices in BBQ sauce.
2. Grill or bake tempeh until heated through.
3. In a bowl, mix cabbage, carrot, vegan mayonnaise, and apple cider vinegar.
4. Season with salt and pepper.
5. Assemble sandwiches with BBQ tempeh and slaw.

Nutrition Information:

- Calories: 280
- Protein: 14g
- Carbohydrates: 30g
- Fat: 12g
- Fiber: 6g
- Sugar: 8g
- Portion Size: 1 sandwich

Chapter 4: Dinner Recipes

Embrace the delightful journey of crafting delectable vegan dinners specially designed for those managing Type 2 Diabetes. Each recipe in this chapter is meticulously curated to balance flavor, nutrition, and simplicity. Let these recipes be a testament to the joy of nourishing your body with wholesome ingredients.

Eggplant and Spinach Lasagna

Ingredients:

- 2 medium-sized eggplants, thinly sliced
- 2 cups fresh spinach, chopped
- 1 cup vegan ricotta cheese
- 2 cups marinara sauce
- 1 cup vegan mozzarella cheese, shredded
- 12 lasagna noodles, cooked al dente
- Salt and pepper to taste
- Olive oil for greasing

Instructions:

1. Preheat the oven to 375°F (190°C).

2. In a pan, sauté the sliced eggplants with salt until tender. Set aside.

3. In a bowl, combine chopped spinach and vegan ricotta cheese.

4. Grease a baking dish and layer it with marinara sauce.

5. Arrange lasagna noodles, followed by a layer of sautéed eggplants and the spinach-ricotta mixture.

6. Repeat the layers and top with vegan mozzarella.

7. Bake for 25-30 minutes until golden.

8. Let it cool before slicing.

Nutrition Information (per serving):

- Calories: 320
- Protein: 14g
- Carbohydrates: 40g
- Fat: 12g
- Fiber: 8g
- Sugar: 10g
- Portion size: 1 slice

Chickpea and Vegetable Stir-Fry

Ingredients:

- 1 can chickpeas, drained and rinsed
- 2 cups mixed vegetables (broccoli, bell peppers, snap peas)
- 1 tablespoon sesame oil
- 3 tablespoons soy sauce
- 1 tablespoon maple syrup
- 1 teaspoon ginger, minced
- 2 cloves garlic, minced
- 2 green onions, chopped
- Sesame seeds for garnish

Instructions:

1. Heat sesame oil in a wok or skillet.
2. Add minced garlic and ginger, sauté until fragrant.
3. Toss in mixed vegetables and chickpeas, stir-fry until crisp-tender.
4. In a bowl, mix soy sauce and maple syrup, then pour over the vegetables.
5. Stir well, ensuring even coating.
6. Garnish with green onions and sesame seeds.

7. Serve over brown rice or quinoa.

Nutrition Information (per serving):

- Calories: 280
- Protein: 12g
- Carbohydrates: 40g
- Fat: 8g
- Fiber: 10g
- Sugar: 8g
- Portion size: 1 cup

Stuffed Acorn Squash with Quinoa

Ingredients:

- 3 acorn squash, halved and seeds removed
- 1 cup quinoa, cooked
- 1 cup black beans, cooked
- 1 cup cherry tomatoes, halved
- 1 cup corn kernels
- 1 teaspoon cumin
- 1 teaspoon chili powder
- Salt and pepper to taste
- Fresh cilantro for garnish

Instructions:

1. Preheat the oven to 400°F (200°C).
2. Place acorn squash halves on a baking sheet.
3. In a bowl, mix cooked quinoa, black beans, cherry tomatoes, corn, cumin, chili powder, salt, and pepper.
4. Stuff each squash half with the quinoa mixture.
5. Bake for 30-35 minutes until squash is tender.
6. Garnish with fresh cilantro before serving.

Nutrition Information (per serving):

- Calories: 340
- Protein: 15g
- Carbohydrates: 60g
- Fat: 5g
- Fiber: 12g
- Sugar: 6g
- Portion size: 1 stuffed half

Vegan Chili with Kidney Beans

Ingredients:

- 2 cans kidney beans, drained and rinsed

- 1 can diced tomatoes

- 1 cup corn kernels

- 1 cup bell peppers, diced

- 1 onion, chopped

- 3 cloves garlic, minced

- 2 tablespoons chili powder

- 1 teaspoon cumin

- Salt and pepper to taste

- Fresh cilantro for garnish

Instructions:

1. In a large pot, sauté onions and garlic until translucent.

2. Add bell peppers, corn, diced tomatoes, kidney beans, chili powder, cumin, salt, and pepper.

3. Simmer for 25-30 minutes.

4. Garnish with fresh cilantro before serving.

Nutrition Information (per serving):

- Calories: 290

- Protein: 14g

- Carbohydrates: 55g

- Fat: 2g

- Fiber: 14g

- Sugar: 8g

- Portion size: 1 cup

Cauliflower and Potato Curry

Ingredients:

- 1 small cauliflower, cut into florets

- 2 potatoes, peeled and diced

- 1 can chickpeas, drained and rinsed

- 1 can coconut milk

- 1 onion, finely chopped

- 3 cloves garlic, minced

- 1 tablespoon curry powder

- 1 teaspoon turmeric

- Salt and pepper to taste

- Fresh cilantro for garnish

Instructions:

1. In a large pan, sauté onions and garlic until golden.

2. Add curry powder, turmeric, cauliflower, potatoes, and chickpeas.

3. Pour in coconut milk and simmer until vegetables are tender.

4. Season with salt and pepper.

5. Garnish with fresh cilantro before serving.

Nutrition Information (per serving):

- Calories: 320

- Protein: 10g

- Carbohydrates: 45g

- Fat: 14g

- Fiber: 10g

- Sugar: 8g

- Portion size: 1 cup

Zoodle (Zucchini Noodle) Alfredo

Ingredients:

- 4 medium zucchinis, spiralized into noodles

- 1 cup cashews, soaked and drained

- 2 cups unsweetened almond milk

- 3 cloves garlic, minced

- 1 tablespoon nutritional yeast

- Salt and pepper to taste

- Fresh parsley for garnish

Instructions:

1. In a blender, combine soaked cashews, almond milk, minced garlic, nutritional yeast, salt, and pepper.
2. Blend until smooth and creamy.
3. In a pan, sauté zucchini noodles until just tender.
4. Pour the Alfredo sauce over the noodles and toss until well-coated.
5. Garnish with fresh parsley before serving.

Nutrition Information (per serving):

- Calories: 280
- Protein: 8g
- Carbohydrates: 20g
- Fat: 18g
- Fiber: 4g
- Sugar: 6g
- Portion size: 1 cup

Mexican Quinoa Casserole

Ingredients:

- 1 cup quinoa, uncooked
- 2 cups black beans, cooked
- 1 cup corn kernels
- 1 cup bell peppers, diced
- 1 can diced tomatoes with green chilies
- 1 teaspoon cumin
- 1 teaspoon chili powder
- Salt and pepper to taste
- 1 cup vegan cheese, shredded
- Fresh cilantro for garnish

Instructions:

1. Cook quinoa according to package instructions.
2. In a large bowl, mix cooked quinoa, black beans, corn, bell peppers, diced tomatoes with green chilies, cumin, chili powder, salt, and pepper.
3. Transfer the mixture to a baking dish and top with vegan cheese.
4. Bake at 375°F (190°C) for 20-25 minutes or until cheese is melted and bubbly.

5. Garnish with fresh cilantro before serving.

Nutrition Information (per serving):

- Calories: 310
- Protein: 14g
- Carbohydrates: 50g
- Fat: 7g
- Fiber: 10g
- Sugar: 5g
- Portion size: 1 cup

Portobello Mushroom Steaks

Ingredients:

- 4 large portobello mushrooms, cleaned and stems removed
- 2 tablespoons balsamic vinegar
- 2 tablespoons soy sauce
- 2 cloves garlic, minced
- 1 teaspoon dried thyme
- Salt and pepper to taste
- Olive oil for brushing

Instructions:

1. In a bowl, whisk together balsamic vinegar, soy sauce, minced garlic, dried thyme, salt, and pepper.
2. Brush the portobello mushrooms with the marinade.
3. Grill or bake the mushrooms for 10-12 minutes, turning once.
4. Serve hot.

Nutrition Information (per serving):

- Calories: 120
- Protein: 8g
- Carbohydrates: 12g
- Fat: 6g
- Fiber: 4g
- Sugar: 4g
- Portion size: 1 mushroom

Ratatouille with Herbed Polenta

Ingredients:

- 1 eggplant, thinly sliced
- 2 zucchinis, thinly sliced
- 1 yellow bell pepper, thinly sliced

- 1 red onion, thinly sliced
- 3 tomatoes, thinly sliced
- 2 cloves garlic, minced
- 2 tablespoons tomato paste
- 1 teaspoon dried oregano
- 1 teaspoon dried basil
- Salt and pepper to taste

Herbed Polenta:
- 1 cup polenta
- 4 cups vegetable broth
- 2 tablespoons vegan butter
- 1 teaspoon dried thyme
- Salt and pepper to taste

Instructions:

1. Preheat the oven to 375°F (190°C).
2. In a baking dish, layer sliced eggplant, zucchini, bell pepper, onion, and tomatoes.
3. Mix minced garlic, tomato paste, oregano, basil, salt, and pepper. Spread over the vegetables.
4. Bake for 45-50 minutes until vegetables are tender.

5. For the herbed polenta, bring vegetable broth to a boil. Whisk in polenta, vegan butter, thyme, salt, and pepper. Cook until thickened.

6. Serve Ratatouille over herbed polenta.

Nutrition Information (per serving):

- Calories: 280
- Protein: 6g
- Carbohydrates: 50g
- Fat: 8g
- Fiber: 10g
- Sugar: 8g
- Portion size: 1 cup Ratatouille with 1/2 cup polenta

Thai Basil Tofu Stir-Fry

Ingredients:

- 1 block firm tofu, pressed and cubed
- 2 tablespoons soy sauce
- 1 tablespoon hoisin sauce
- 1 tablespoon maple syrup
- 1 tablespoon vegetable oil
- 1 bell pepper, sliced

- 1 cup snap peas

- 1 carrot, julienned

- 3 green onions, chopped

- 1 tablespoon fresh basil, chopped

- Cooked brown rice for serving

Instructions:

1. In a bowl, mix cubed tofu with soy sauce, hoisin sauce, and maple syrup. Marinate for 15 minutes.
2. Heat vegetable oil in a wok or skillet. Add marinated tofu and stir-fry until golden.
3. Add sliced bell pepper, snap peas, carrot, and green onions. Stir-fry for an additional 5 minutes.
4. Sprinkle fresh basil over the stir-fry.
5. Serve over cooked brown rice.

Nutrition Information (per serving):

- Calories: 320

- Protein: 16g

- Carbohydrates: 40g

- Fat: 12g

- Fiber: 8g

- Sugar: 10g
- Portion size: 1 cup

Wild Rice and Vegetable Pilaf

Ingredients:

- 1 cup wild rice, cooked
- 1 cup mixed vegetables (peas, carrots, corn)
- 1 cup mushrooms, sliced
- 1 onion, chopped
- 2 cloves garlic, minced
- 2 tablespoons olive oil
- 1 teaspoon thyme
- Salt and pepper to taste
- 1/4 cup almonds, toasted
- Fresh parsley for garnish

Instructions:

1. In a pan, sauté onions and garlic in olive oil until softened.
2. Add sliced mushrooms and cook until browned.
3. Stir in mixed vegetables and cooked wild rice. Cook until heated through.

4. Season with thyme, salt, and pepper.

5. Garnish with toasted almonds and fresh parsley before serving.

Nutrition Information (per serving):

- Calories: 290
- Protein: 10g
- Carbohydrates: 35g
- Fat: 14g
- Fiber: 6g
- Sugar: 4g
- Portion size: 1 cup

Spiced Lentil and Vegetable Skewers

Ingredients:

- 1 cup dry lentils, cooked
- 1 zucchini, cut into chunks
- 1 bell pepper, cut into chunks
- 1 red onion, cut into chunks
- 2 tablespoons olive oil

- 1 teaspoon cumin
- 1 teaspoon paprika
- 1 teaspoon coriander
- Salt and pepper to taste
- Lemon wedges for serving

Instructions:

1. In a bowl, mix cooked lentils, zucchini, bell pepper, red onion, olive oil, cumin, paprika, coriander, salt, and pepper.
2. Thread the mixture onto skewers.
3. Grill or bake for 15-20 minutes until vegetables are tender.
4. Serve with lemon wedges.

Nutrition Information (per serving):

- Calories: 250
- Protein: 15g
- Carbohydrates: 35g
- Fat: 6g
- Fiber: 12g
- Sugar: 6g

- Portion size: 1 skewer

Creamy Mushroom and Spinach Risotto

Ingredients:

- 1 cup Arborio rice
- 4 cups vegetable broth, heated
- 1 cup mushrooms, sliced
- 2 cups fresh spinach
- 1 onion, finely chopped
- 2 cloves garlic, minced
- 1/2 cup dry white wine
- 2 tablespoons nutritional yeast
- 2 tablespoons vegan butter
- Salt and pepper to taste
- Fresh parsley for garnish

Instructions:

1. In a pan, sauté onions and garlic in vegan butter until translucent.
2. Add Arborio rice and cook for 2 minutes.

3. Pour in white wine and simmer until mostly evaporated.

4. Begin adding hot vegetable broth, one ladle at a time, stirring continuously until absorbed.

5. Continue until rice is creamy and cooked al dente.

6. Stir in sliced mushrooms, fresh spinach, nutritional yeast, salt, and pepper.

7. Garnish with fresh parsley before serving.

Nutrition Information (per serving):

- Calories: 320
- Protein: 8g
- Carbohydrates: 55g
- Fat: 8g
- Fiber: 6g
- Sugar: 4g
- Portion size: 1 cup

Vegan Jambalaya with Okra

Ingredients:

- 1 cup brown rice, uncooked
- 1 can kidney beans, drained and rinsed

- 1 cup okra, sliced

- 1 bell pepper, diced

- 1 onion, chopped

- 2 cloves garlic, minced

- 1 can diced tomatoes

- 1 teaspoon smoked paprika

- 1 teaspoon thyme

- 1/2 teaspoon cayenne pepper

- Salt and pepper to taste

- Fresh parsley for garnish

Instructions:

1. Cook brown rice according to package instructions.

2. In a large pot, sauté onions and garlic until softened.

3. Add diced bell pepper, okra, kidney beans, diced tomatoes, smoked paprika, thyme, cayenne pepper, salt, and pepper.

4. Simmer for 20-25 minutes.

5. Serve over cooked brown rice.

6. Garnish with fresh parsley.

Nutrition Information (per serving):

- Calories: 280
- Protein: 12g
- Carbohydrates: 50g
- Fat: 4g
- Fiber: 10g
- Sugar: 6g
- Portion size: 1 cup

Butternut Squash and Sage Risotto

Ingredients:

- 1 cup Arborio rice
- 4 cups vegetable broth, heated
- 2 cups butternut squash, diced
- 1 onion, finely chopped
- 2 cloves garlic, minced
- 1/2 cup dry white wine
- 2 tablespoons nutritional yeast
- 2 tablespoons vegan butter
- Salt and pepper to taste
- Fresh sage leaves for garnish

Instructions:

1. In a pan, sauté onions and garlic in vegan butter until translucent.
2. Add Arborio rice and cook for 2 minutes.
3. Pour in white wine and simmer until mostly evaporated.
4. Begin adding hot vegetable broth, one ladle at a time, stirring continuously until absorbed.
5. Continue until rice is creamy and cooked al dente.
6. Stir in diced butternut squash, nutritional yeast, salt, and pepper.
7. Garnish with fresh sage leaves before serving.

Nutrition Information (per serving):

- Calories: 300
- Protein: 6g
- Carbohydrates: 60g
- Fat: 6g
- Fiber: 8g
- Sugar: 4g
- Portion size: 1 cup

Chapter 5: Snacks and Appetizers

These vegan treats are not only satisfying to the taste buds but are also curated to support a balanced and healthy lifestyle. Explore the array of colors, textures, and tastes that await you in this chapter, where each recipe is a testament to the delicious possibilities of diabetic-friendly, vegan cuisine.

Guacamole with Veggie Sticks

Ingredients:

- 3 ripe avocados
- 1 small red onion, finely diced
- 2 tomatoes, diced
- 1 clove garlic, minced
- 1 lime, juiced
- Salt and pepper to taste
- Assorted veggie sticks for dipping (carrots, cucumbers, bell peppers)

Instructions:

1. Mash avocados in a bowl.

2. Add diced red onion, tomatoes, minced garlic, and lime juice.

3. Season with salt and pepper, mix well.

4. Chill in the refrigerator for 30 minutes.

5. Serve with veggie sticks.

Nutrition Information (per serving):

- Calories: 120
- Protein: 2g
- Carbohydrates: 8g
- Fat: 10g
- Fiber: 5g
- Sugar: 1g
- Portion Size: 1/4 cup guacamole with veggie sticks

Roasted Red Pepper Hummus

Ingredients:

- 1 can (15 oz) chickpeas, drained and rinsed
- 2 roasted red peppers
- 3 tbsp tahini
- 2 cloves garlic
- 2 tbsp lemon juice

- 1/4 cup olive oil

- Salt and cumin to taste

Instructions:

1. Combine chickpeas, roasted red peppers, tahini, garlic, and lemon juice in a food processor.
2. Blend while drizzling in olive oil until smooth.
3. Season with salt and cumin to taste.
4. Refrigerate before serving.

Nutrition Information (per serving):

- Calories: 150

- Protein: 5g

- Carbohydrates: 12g

- Fat: 10g

- Fiber: 4g

- Sugar: 2g

- Portion Size: 2 tbsp hummus

Vegan Spinach and Artichoke Dip

Ingredients:

- 1 cup frozen chopped spinach, thawed and drained

- 1 can (14 oz) artichoke hearts, chopped

- 1 cup vegan cream cheese

- 1/2 cup vegan mayonnaise

- 1 cup vegan shredded mozzarella

- 2 cloves garlic, minced

- Salt and pepper to taste

Instructions:

1. Preheat oven to 350°F (175°C).

2. In a bowl, mix spinach, artichoke hearts, vegan cream cheese, vegan mayonnaise, vegan shredded mozzarella, and minced garlic.

3. Season with salt and pepper.

4. Transfer to a baking dish and bake for 25 minutes.

5. Serve warm.

Nutrition Information (per serving):

- Calories: 180

- Protein: 4g

- Carbohydrates: 8g

- Fat: 15g

- Fiber: 2g

- Sugar: 1g
- Portion Size: 1/4 cup dip

Edamame and Sesame Seed Crackers

Ingredients:

- 1 cup shelled edamame, cooked
- 1 cup almond flour
- 2 tbsp sesame seeds
- 1 tbsp nutritional yeast
- 1 tsp garlic powder
- Salt to taste
- Water as needed

Instructions:

1. Preheat oven to 350°F (175°C).
2. In a food processor, combine edamame, almond flour, sesame seeds, nutritional yeast, garlic powder, and a pinch of salt.
3. Pulse until a dough forms, adding water if needed.

4. Roll out the dough between parchment papers, then cut into crackers.

5. Bake for 12-15 minutes or until golden brown.

Nutrition Information (per serving):

- Calories: 90
- Protein: 5g
- Carbohydrates: 5g
- Fat: 5g
- Fiber: 2g
- Sugar: 1g
- Portion Size: 6 crackers

Spicy Avocado Salsa

Ingredients:

- 2 ripe avocados, diced
- 1 cup cherry tomatoes, halved
- 1/4 cup red onion, finely chopped
- 1 jalapeño, minced (seeds removed for less heat)
- 1/4 cup fresh cilantro, chopped
- 1 lime, juiced
- Salt and pepper to taste

Instructions:

1. In a bowl, combine diced avocados, cherry tomatoes, red onion, jalapeño, and cilantro.
2. Drizzle lime juice over the mixture and gently toss.
3. Season with salt and pepper.
4. Refrigerate for 20 minutes before serving.

Nutrition Information (per serving):

- Calories: 110
- Protein: 2g
- Carbohydrates: 8g
- Fat: 9g
- Fiber: 5g
- Sugar: 1g
- Portion Size: 1/2 cup salsa

Baked Sweet Potato Fries

Ingredients:

- 2 large sweet potatoes, cut into fries
- 2 tbsp olive oil
- 1 tsp paprika
- 1/2 tsp garlic powder

- 1/2 tsp onion powder
- Salt and pepper to taste

Instructions:

1. Preheat oven to 425°F (220°C).
2. In a bowl, toss sweet potato fries with olive oil, paprika, garlic powder, onion powder, salt, and pepper.
3. Spread fries on a baking sheet in a single layer.
4. Bake for 25-30 minutes, flipping halfway through.

Nutrition Information (per serving):

- Calories: 120
- Protein: 2g
- Carbohydrates: 20g
- Fat: 4g
- Fiber: 4g
- Sugar: 4g
- Portion Size: 1 cup fries

Stuffed Grape Leaves with Tofu

Ingredients:

- 1 jar grape leaves, drained
- 1 cup firm tofu, crumbled
- 1/2 cup cooked quinoa
- 1/4 cup pine nuts
- 2 tbsp fresh dill, chopped
- 2 tbsp lemon juice
- Salt and pepper to taste

Instructions:

1. Mix crumbled tofu, cooked quinoa, pine nuts, dill, and lemon juice in a bowl.
2. Place a grape leaf flat, spoon mixture onto the center, and fold to enclose.
3. Repeat with remaining leaves.
4. Steam for 15 minutes.
5. Allow to cool before serving.

Nutrition Information (per serving):

- Calories: 130
- Protein: 6g

- Carbohydrates: 10g

- Fat: 8g

- Fiber: 2g

- Sugar: 0g

- Portion Size: 4 stuffed grape leaves

Vegan Caprese Skewers

Ingredients:

- 1 pint cherry tomatoes

- 1 cup vegan mozzarella, cubed

- Fresh basil leaves

- Balsamic glaze for drizzling

- Wooden skewers

Instructions:

1. Thread a tomato, a cube of vegan mozzarella, and a basil leaf onto each skewer.

2. Arrange on a serving platter.

3. Drizzle with balsamic glaze before serving.

Nutrition Information (per serving):

- Calories: 90

- Protein: 5g

- Carbohydrates: 5g

- Fat: 5g

- Fiber: 1g

- Sugar: 2g

- Portion Size: 3 skewers

Kale Chips with Nutritional Yeast

Ingredients:

- 1 bunch kale, stems removed and torn into pieces

- 2 tbsp olive oil

- 2 tbsp nutritional yeast

- Salt to taste

Instructions:

1. Preheat oven to 300°F (150°C).

2. Massage kale with olive oil until coated.

3. Sprinkle nutritional yeast and salt, tossing to coat.

4. Spread on a baking sheet and bake for 15-20 minutes or until crisp.

Nutrition Information (per serving):

- Calories: 60
- Protein: 3g
- Carbohydrates: 5g
- Fat: 4g
- Fiber: 2g
- Sugar: 0g
- Portion Size: 1 cup kale chips

Buffalo Cauliflower Bites

Ingredients:

- 1 head cauliflower, cut into florets
- 1/2 cup almond flour
- 1/2 cup unsweetened almond milk
- 1 tsp garlic powder
- 1 tsp onion powder
- 1/2 cup buffalo sauce

Instructions:

1. Preheat oven to 450°F (230°C).
2. In a bowl, mix almond flour, almond milk, garlic powder, and onion powder to form a batter.

3. Dip cauliflower florets into the batter, then place on a baking sheet.

4. Bake for 20 minutes, tossing halfway.

5. Toss with buffalo sauce before serving.

Nutrition Information (per serving):

- Calories: 120
- Protein: 5g
- Carbohydrates: 15g
- Fat: 5g
- Fiber: 5g
- Sugar: 2g
- Portion Size: 1 cup cauliflower bites

Vegan Cheese and Crackers

Ingredients:

- 1 cup vegan cheese, sliced or shredded
- 1 cup whole grain crackers
- Fresh herbs for garnish (optional)

Instructions:

1. Arrange vegan cheese slices or shreds on a serving
    platter.
2. Place whole grain crackers around the cheese.
3. Garnish with fresh herbs if desired.
4. Serve at room temperature.

Nutrition Information (per serving):

- Calories: 160
- Protein: 5g
- Carbohydrates: 20g
- Fat: 8g
- Fiber: 4g
- Sugar: 1g
- Portion Size: 6 crackers with cheese

Avocado and Black Bean Salsa

Ingredients:

- 2 ripe avocados, diced
- 1 can (15 oz) black beans, drained and rinsed
- 1 cup corn kernels (fresh or frozen)
- 1/4 cup red onion, finely chopped

- 1/4 cup cilantro, chopped

- 2 tbsp lime juice

- Salt and cumin to taste

Instructions:

1. In a bowl, combine diced avocados, black beans, corn, red onion, and cilantro.
2. Drizzle lime juice over the mixture and gently toss.
3. Season with salt and cumin.
4. Refrigerate for 30 minutes before serving.

Nutrition Information (per serving):

- Calories: 150

- Protein: 6g

- Carbohydrates: 20g

- Fat: 6g

- Fiber: 8g

- Sugar: 2g

- Portion Size: 1/2 cup salsa

Almond and Cranberry Energy Bites

Ingredients:

- 1 cup rolled oats
- 1/2 cup almond butter
- 1/4 cup maple syrup
- 1/4 cup dried cranberries, chopped
- 1/4 cup almonds, chopped
- 1 tsp vanilla extract
- A pinch of salt

Instructions:

1. In a bowl, mix rolled oats, almond butter, maple syrup, dried cranberries, almonds, vanilla extract, and a pinch of salt.
2. Form into bite-sized balls.
3. Refrigerate for at least 1 hour before serving.

Nutrition Information (per serving):

- Calories: 100
- Protein: 3g
- Carbohydrates: 12g
- Fat: 5g

- Fiber: 2g

- Sugar: 5g

- Portion Size: 2 energy bites

Cucumber Rolls with Vegan Cream Cheese

Ingredients:

- 2 large cucumbers, thinly sliced lengthwise

- 1 cup vegan cream cheese

- 1/4 cup sun-dried tomatoes, chopped

- Fresh basil leaves

Instructions:

1. Lay cucumber slices flat and spread a layer of vegan cream cheese on each.

2. Sprinkle sun-dried tomatoes on the cream cheese.

3. Place a fresh basil leaf on one end and roll the cucumber slice.

4. Secure with a toothpick if needed.

Nutrition Information (per serving):

- Calories: 80
- Protein: 2g
- Carbohydrates: 5g
- Fat: 6g
- Fiber: 1g
- Sugar: 2g
- Portion Size: 4 cucumber rolls

Roasted Chickpeas with Smoky Paprika

Ingredients:

- 1 can (15 oz) chickpeas, drained and dried
- 1 tbsp olive oil
- 1 tsp smoked paprika
- 1/2 tsp garlic powder
- 1/2 tsp cumin
- Salt to taste

Instructions:

1. Preheat oven to 400°F (200°C).

2. Toss dried chickpeas with olive oil, smoked paprika, garlic powder, cumin, and salt.

3. Spread on a baking sheet and roast for 20-25 minutes until crunchy.

Nutrition Information (per serving):

- Calories: 120
- Protein: 5g
- Carbohydrates: 15g
- Fat: 5g
- Fiber: 4g
- Sugar: 3g
- Portion Size: 1/2 cup roasted chickpeas

Chapter 6: Desserts

These dessert recipes are crafted with wholesome ingredients, striking the perfect balance between flavor and nutritional goodness. From tantalizing tarts to guilt-free mousse, each treat is a testament to the joy of savoring sweetness responsibly. So, let's embark on a delightful journey through these diabetic-friendly desserts.

Berry and Almond Tart

Ingredients:

- 1 cup fresh mixed berries (strawberries, blueberries, raspberries)
- 1 cup almond flour
- 2 tablespoons coconut oil, melted
- 2 tablespoons maple syrup
- 1 teaspoon vanilla extract
- Pinch of salt

Instructions:

1. Preheat oven to 350°F (175°C).

2. In a bowl, mix almond flour, melted coconut oil, maple syrup, vanilla extract, and a pinch of salt.

3. Press the mixture into a tart pan to form a crust.

4. Bake for 10 minutes or until the edges are golden brown.

5. Allow the crust to cool, then fill with fresh mixed berries.

Nutrition Information (per serving):

- Calories: 180
- Protein: 4g
- Carbohydrates: 14g
- Fat: 12g
- Fiber: 3g
- Sugar: 8g
- Portion Size: 1 slice

Vegan Chocolate Avocado Mousse

Ingredients:

- 2 ripe avocados
- 1/4 cup cocoa powder
- 1/4 cup maple syrup

- 1 teaspoon vanilla extract

- Pinch of salt

- 1/4 cup almond milk

Instructions:

1. Blend avocados, cocoa powder, maple syrup, vanilla extract, and salt until smooth.

2. Add almond milk gradually until desired consistency is achieved.

3. Refrigerate for at least 2 hours before serving.

Nutrition Information (per serving):

- Calories: 200

- Protein: 3g

- Carbohydrates: 15g

- Fat: 15g

- Fiber: 7g

- Sugar: 5g

- Portion Size: 1/2 cup

Pumpkin Pie with Oat Crust

Ingredients:

- 1 can (15 oz) pumpkin puree
- 1/2 cup oat flour
- 1/2 cup rolled oats
- 1/4 cup coconut oil, melted
- 1/4 cup maple syrup
- 1 teaspoon pumpkin spice blend
- 1/2 teaspoon vanilla extract

Instructions:

1. Preheat oven to 350°F (175°C).
2. Mix oat flour, rolled oats, melted coconut oil, maple syrup, pumpkin spice, and vanilla extract to form the crust.
3. Press the crust into a pie pan.
4. In a separate bowl, mix pumpkin puree and pour into the crust.
5. Bake for 40-45 minutes.

Nutrition Information (per serving):

- Calories: 220

- Protein: 3g

- Carbohydrates: 20g

- Fat: 14g

- Fiber: 5g

- Sugar: 8g

- Portion Size: 1 slice

Coconut and Lime Sorbet

Ingredients:

- 2 cans (28 oz) coconut milk

- Zest and juice of 3 limes

- 1/2 cup agave syrup

- 1 teaspoon vanilla extract

Instructions:

1. Blend coconut milk, lime zest, lime juice, agave syrup, and vanilla extract until smooth.

2. Pour the mixture into an ice cream maker and churn according to the manufacturer's instructions.

3. Transfer to a lidded container and freeze for at least 4 hours before serving.

Nutrition Information (per serving):

- Calories: 180
- Protein: 1g
- Carbohydrates: 15g
- Fat: 14g
- Fiber: 2g
- Sugar: 10g
- Portion Size: 1/2 cup

Apple Cinnamon Baked Oatmeal

Ingredients:

- 2 cups rolled oats
- 1 1/2 cups unsweetened almond milk
- 2 apples, peeled and diced
- 1/4 cup maple syrup
- 1 teaspoon cinnamon
- 1/4 cup chopped nuts (walnuts or almonds)

Instructions:

1. Preheat oven to 350°F (175°C).
2. In a bowl, mix rolled oats, almond milk, diced apples, maple syrup, and cinnamon.

3. Transfer the mixture to a baking dish and sprinkle chopped nuts on top.

4. Bake for 30-35 minutes until the oats are set.

5. Allow to cool before serving.

Nutrition Information (per serving):

- Calories: 220

- Protein: 5g

- Carbohydrates: 35g

- Fat: 6g

- Fiber: 6g

- Sugar: 14g

- Portion Size: 1 square

Chocolate Chip Banana Bread

Ingredients:

- 3 ripe bananas, mashed

- 1/4 cup coconut oil, melted

- 1/4 cup maple syrup

- 1 teaspoon vanilla extract

- 2 cups whole wheat flour

- 1 teaspoon baking soda

- 1/2 teaspoon salt
- 1/2 cup vegan chocolate chips

Instructions:

1. Preheat oven to 350°F (175°C).
2. In a bowl, mix mashed bananas, melted coconut oil, maple syrup, and vanilla extract.
3. In a separate bowl, combine whole wheat flour, baking soda, and salt.
4. Gradually add the dry ingredients to the wet ingredients and mix until well combined.
5. Fold in the chocolate chips.
6. Transfer the batter to a greased loaf pan and bake for 50-60 minutes.

Nutrition Information (per serving):

- Calories: 180
- Protein: 3g
- Carbohydrates: 28g
- Fat: 7g
- Fiber: 4g
- Sugar: 12g

- Portion Size: 1 slice

Vegan Lemon Bars

Ingredients:

- 1 cup almond flour
- 1/4 cup coconut flour
- 1/4 cup coconut oil, melted
- 1/4 cup maple syrup
- Zest and juice of 2 lemons
- 1/4 cup arrowroot powder
- 1/2 cup coconut milk

Instructions:

1. Preheat oven to 350°F (175°C).
2. In a bowl, mix almond flour, coconut flour, melted coconut oil, and maple syrup.
3. Press the mixture into a baking dish to form the crust and bake for 10 minutes.
4. In another bowl, whisk together lemon zest, lemon juice, arrowroot powder, and coconut milk.
5. Pour the lemon mixture over the crust and bake for an additional 20 minutes.

6. Allow to cool before cutting into bars.

Nutrition Information (per serving):

- Calories: 160
- Protein: 2g
- Carbohydrates: 15g
- Fat: 10g
- Fiber: 2g
- Sugar: 6g
- Portion Size: 1 bar

Raspberry Chia Seed Pudding

Ingredients:

- 1/2 cup chia seeds
- 2 cups almond milk
- 1 cup fresh raspberries
- 2 tablespoons maple syrup
- 1/2 teaspoon vanilla extract

Instructions:

1. In a bowl, mix chia seeds, almond milk, maple syrup, and vanilla extract.

2. Let it sit in the refrigerator for at least 4 hours or overnight.

3. Before serving, layer chia pudding with fresh raspberries.

Nutrition Information (per serving):

- Calories: 180

- Protein: 5g

- Carbohydrates: 20g

- Fat: 9g

- Fiber: 10g

- Sugar: 8g

- Portion Size: 1/2 cup

Almond Butter and Jelly Thumbprint Cookies

Ingredients:

- 1 cup almond flour

- 1/4 cup almond butter

- 1/4 cup maple syrup

- 1/4 cup fruit-sweetened jam (raspberry, strawberry, or your choice)

Instructions:

1. Preheat oven to 350°F (175°C).
2. In a bowl, mix almond flour, almond butter, and maple syrup.
3. Form small balls and place them on a baking sheet.
4. Make a thumbprint in the center of each cookie and fill with a small spoonful of jam.
5. Bake for 10-12 minutes.

Nutrition Information (per serving):

- Calories: 120
- Protein: 3g
- Carbohydrates: 12g
- Fat: 7g
- Fiber: 2g
- Sugar: 6g
- Portion Size: 2 cookies

Dark Chocolate Covered Strawberries

Ingredients:

- 1 cup dark chocolate chips
- 1 pound fresh strawberries, washed and dried

Instructions:

1. Melt dark chocolate chips in a heatproof bowl over simmering water or in the microwave.
2. Dip each strawberry into the melted chocolate, ensuring it's coated.
3. Place on a parchment-lined tray and refrigerate until the chocolate hardens.

Nutrition Information (per serving):

- Calories: 120
- Protein: 1g
- Carbohydrates: 15g
- Fat: 7g
- Fiber: 3g
- Sugar: 10g
- Portion Size: 4 strawberries

Blueberry and Lemon Coconut Bliss Balls

Ingredients:

- 1 cup dried blueberries
- 1 cup shredded coconut
- Zest and juice of 1 lemon
- 1/4 cup almond flour
- 2 tablespoons maple syrup

Instructions:

1. In a food processor, combine dried blueberries, shredded coconut, lemon zest, lemon juice, almond flour, and maple syrup.
2. Pulse until the mixture forms a sticky dough.
3. Roll the dough into bite-sized balls and refrigerate for at least 1 hour before serving.

Nutrition Information (per serving):

- Calories: 130
- Protein: 2g
- Carbohydrates: 18g
- Fat: 6g

- Fiber: 3g

- Sugar: 10g

- Portion Size: 2 balls

Pistachio and Cranberry Biscotti

Ingredients:

- 2 cups whole wheat flour

- 1/2 cup maple syrup

- 1/4 cup coconut oil, melted

- 1/2 cup shelled pistachios, chopped

- 1/2 cup dried cranberries

- 1 teaspoon baking powder

- 1/4 teaspoon salt

Instructions:

1. Preheat oven to 350°F (175°C).

2. In a bowl, mix whole wheat flour, maple syrup, melted coconut oil, chopped pistachios, dried cranberries, baking powder, and salt.

3. Form the dough into two logs on a baking sheet and bake for 20-25 minutes.

4. Slice the logs into biscotti and bake for an additional 10 minutes.

Nutrition Information (per serving):

- Calories: 160
- Protein: 3g
- Carbohydrates: 22g
- Fat: 7g
- Fiber: 2g
- Sugar: 10g
- Portion Size: 2 biscotti

Mango and Coconut Rice Pudding

Ingredients:

- 1 cup arborio rice
- 2 cups coconut milk
- 1 cup diced mango
- 1/4 cup maple syrup
- 1/2 teaspoon vanilla extract
- Pinch of salt

Instructions:

1. In a saucepan, combine arborio rice, coconut milk, diced mango, maple syrup, vanilla extract, and a pinch of salt.
2. Bring to a simmer, then reduce heat and let it cook until the rice is tender and the mixture thickens.
3. Remove from heat and let it cool before serving.

Nutrition Information (per serving):

- Calories: 200
- Protein: 3g
- Carbohydrates: 35g
- Fat: 6g
- Fiber: 2g
- Sugar: 15g
- Portion Size: 1/2 cup

Chocolate Peanut Butter Cupcakes

Ingredients:

- 1 cup whole wheat flour
- 1/2 cup cocoa powder
- 1 teaspoon baking powder

- 1/2 teaspoon baking soda

- 1/4 cup coconut oil, melted

- 1/2 cup maple syrup

- 1/2 cup unsweetened applesauce

- 1/4 cup peanut butter

Instructions:

1. Preheat oven to 350°F (175°C).

2. In a bowl, mix whole wheat flour, cocoa powder, baking powder, and baking soda.

3. In another bowl, combine melted coconut oil, maple syrup, applesauce, and peanut butter.

4. Gradually add the dry ingredients to the wet ingredients and mix until well combined.

5. Spoon the batter into cupcake liners and bake for 20-25 minutes.

Nutrition Information (per serving):

- Calories: 180

- Protein: 4g

- Carbohydrates: 25g

- Fat: 8g

- Fiber: 3g
- Sugar: 10g
- Portion Size: 1 cupcake

Avocado Chocolate Mousse Tart

Ingredients:

- 1 cup almond flour
- 1/4 cup cocoa powder
- 1/4 cup coconut oil, melted
- 1/4 cup maple syrup
- 2 ripe avocados
- 1/4 cup cocoa powder
- 1/4 cup coconut milk
- 1/4 cup maple syrup
- 1 teaspoon vanilla extract

Instructions:

1. Preheat oven to 350°F (175°C).
2. In a bowl, mix almond flour, cocoa powder, melted coconut oil, and maple syrup to form the crust.
3. Press the crust into a tart pan and bake for 10 minutes.

4. In a blender, combine ripe avocados, cocoa powder, coconut milk, maple syrup, and vanilla extract until smooth.

5. Pour the avocado chocolate mousse into the tart crust and refrigerate for at least 2 hours before serving.

Nutrition Information (per serving):

- Calories: 190

- Protein: 3g

- Carbohydrates: 20g

- Fat: 12g

- Fiber: 5g

- Sugar: 10g

- Portion Size: 1 slice

Chapter 7: Smoothies

Embark on a journey of vibrant flavors and nourishment with our delightful collection of smoothie recipes in Chapter 7. Each concoction is a symphony of wholesome ingredients designed to tantalize your taste buds while providing essential nutrients. Dive into the world of nutritious sips and elevate your well-being with every delicious gulp.

Green Detox Smoothie

Ingredients:

- 1 cup kale leaves, stems removed
- 1/2 cucumber, peeled and sliced
- 1 green apple, cored and chopped
- 1/2 lemon, juiced
- 1 cup coconut water
- Ice cubes (optional)

Instructions:

1. Combine kale, cucumber, green apple, and lemon juice in a blender.

2. Add coconut water and blend until smooth.

3. Add ice cubes if desired and blend again until well combined.

4. Pour into a glass and enjoy!

Nutrition Information:

- Calories: 120
- Protein: 3g
- Carbohydrates: 28g
- Fat: 1g
- Fiber: 5g
- Sugar: 15g
- Portion Size: 1 serving

Berry Blast Smoothie

Ingredients:

- 1 cup mixed berries (strawberries, blueberries, raspberries)
- 1 banana, peeled
- 1/2 cup almond milk
- 1 tablespoon chia seeds
- 1 teaspoon honey (optional)

Instructions:

1. Combine mixed berries, banana, almond milk, and chia seeds in a blender.

2. Add honey if desired and blend until smooth.

3. Pour into a glass and savor the berry bliss!

Nutrition Information:

- Calories: 150

- Protein: 4g

- Carbohydrates: 32g

- Fat: 2g

- Fiber: 8g

- Sugar: 18g

- Portion Size: 1 serving

Tropical Paradise Smoothie

Ingredients:

- 1/2 cup pineapple chunks

- 1/2 cup mango chunks

- 1 banana, peeled

- 1/2 cup coconut water

- 1/4 cup Greek yogurt (vegan if desired)

Instructions:

1. Combine pineapple, mango, banana, coconut water, and Greek yogurt in a blender.
2. Blend until creamy and luscious.
3. Pour into a tropical-themed glass and transport yourself to paradise!

Nutrition Information:

- Calories: 180
- Protein: 5g
- Carbohydrates: 40g
- Fat: 1g
- Fiber: 6g
- Sugar: 25g
- Portion Size: 1 serving

Mango and Spinach Smoothie

Ingredients:

- 1 cup fresh spinach leaves
- 1 cup mango chunks
- 1/2 cup orange juice
- 1/2 cup water

- 1 tablespoon flaxseeds

Instructions:

1. Combine spinach, mango, orange juice, water, and flaxseeds in a blender.
2. Blend until smooth and velvety.
3. Pour into a glass and relish the fusion of mango and greens!

Nutrition Information:

- Calories: 160
- Protein: 4g
- Carbohydrates: 36g
- Fat: 2g
- Fiber: 7g
- Sugar: 25g
- Portion Size: 1 serving

Anti-Inflammatory Turmeric Smoothie

Ingredients:

- 1 cup frozen pineapple chunks
- 1/2 teaspoon turmeric powder
- 1/2 teaspoon ginger, grated
- 1 cup coconut milk
- 1 tablespoon hemp seeds

Instructions:

1. Combine frozen pineapple, turmeric powder, ginger, coconut milk, and hemp seeds in a blender.
2. Blend until the golden elixir is smooth and creamy.
3. Pour into a glass and enjoy the anti-inflammatory goodness!

Nutrition Information:

- Calories: 140
- Protein: 3g
- Carbohydrates: 28g
- Fat: 4g
- Fiber: 5g

- Sugar: 15g
- Portion Size: 1 serving

Blueberry and Almond Butter Smoothie

Ingredients:

- 1 cup blueberries
- 1 tablespoon almond butter
- 1/2 banana, peeled
- 1 cup almond milk
- Ice cubes (optional)

Instructions:

1. Combine blueberries, almond butter, banana, and almond milk in a blender.
2. Add ice cubes if desired and blend until smooth.
3. Pour into a glass and relish the nutty blueberry goodness!

Nutrition Information:

- Calories: 170

- Protein: 4g

- Carbohydrates: 32g

- Fat: 5g

- Fiber: 7g

- Sugar: 18g

- Portion Size: 1 serving

Pineapple Coconut Protein Smoothie

Ingredients:

- 1/2 cup pineapple chunks

- 1/2 cup coconut milk

- 1 scoop vegan protein powder

- 1 tablespoon shredded coconut

- 1/2 teaspoon vanilla extract

Instructions:

1. Combine pineapple, coconut milk, protein powder, shredded coconut, and vanilla extract in a blender.

2. Blend until creamy and protein-packed.

3. Pour into a glass and sip on the tropical protein delight!

Nutrition Information:

- Calories: 200
- Protein: 15g
- Carbohydrates: 25g
- Fat: 8g
- Fiber: 4g
- Sugar: 15g
- Portion Size: 1 serving

Kiwi and Kale Smoothie

Ingredients:

- 2 kiwis, peeled and sliced
- 1 cup kale leaves, stems removed
- 1/2 banana, peeled
- 1/2 cup coconut water
- 1 tablespoon chia seeds

Instructions:

1. Combine kiwis, kale, banana, coconut water, and chia seeds in a blender.
2. Blend until smooth and green perfection is achieved.

3. Pour into a glass and enjoy the nutritional dance of kiwi and kale!

Nutrition Information:

- Calories: 140
- Protein: 4g
- Carbohydrates: 30g
- Fat: 3g
- Fiber: 8g
- Sugar: 15g
- Portion Size: 1 serving

Golden Milk Turmeric Latte Smoothie

Ingredients:

- 1/2 cup frozen mango chunks
- 1/2 teaspoon turmeric powder
- 1/2 teaspoon cinnamon
- 1 cup almond milk
- 1 tablespoon flaxseeds

Instructions:

1. Combine frozen mango, turmeric powder, cinnamon, almond milk, and flaxseeds in a blender.

2. Blend until the golden latte perfection is achieved.

3. Pour into a glass and savor the warmth of golden milk in a smoothie!

Nutrition Information:

- Calories: 160

- Protein: 4g

- Carbohydrates: 32g

- Fat: 4g

- Fiber: 6g

- Sugar: 20g

- Portion Size: 1 serving

Papaya and Lime Smoothie

Ingredients:

- 1 cup papaya chunks

- Juice of 1 lime

- 1/2 cup coconut water

- 1/2 cup water

* 1 tablespoon hemp seeds

Instructions:

1. Combine papaya, lime juice, coconut water, water, and hemp seeds in a blender.
2. Blend until the tropical fusion is smooth and citrusy.
3. Pour into a glass and enjoy the zesty papaya and lime dance!

Nutrition Information:

* Calories: 140
* Protein: 3g
* Carbohydrates: 30g
* Fat: 3g
* Fiber: 6g
* Sugar: 18g
* Portion Size: 1 serving

Peach and Mint Smoothie

Ingredients:

* 1 cup peach slices
* A handful of fresh mint leaves

- 1/2 banana, peeled
- 1/2 cup almond milk
- Ice cubes (optional)

Instructions:

1. Combine peaches, mint leaves, banana, and almond milk in a blender.
2. Add ice cubes if desired and blend until the minty peach delight is achieved.
3. Pour into a glass and revel in the refreshing flavor!

Nutrition Information:

- Calories: 150
- Protein: 3g
- Carbohydrates: 34g
- Fat: 2g
- Fiber: 5g
- Sugar: 20g
- Portion Size: 1 serving

Chocolate Peanut Butter Protein Smoothie

Ingredients:

- 1 tablespoon cocoa powder
- 2 tablespoons peanut butter
- 1 banana, peeled
- 1 cup almond milk
- 1 scoop vegan chocolate protein powder

Instructions:

1. Combine cocoa powder, peanut butter, banana, almond milk, and chocolate protein powder in a blender.
2. Blend until the chocolatey protein goodness is achieved.
3. Pour into a glass and indulge in the decadent treat!

Nutrition Information:

- Calories: 220
- Protein: 20g
- Carbohydrates: 26g
- Fat: 10g

- Fiber: 6g
- Sugar: 15g
- Portion Size: 1 serving

Mixed Berry Chia Seed Smoothie

Ingredients:

- 1 cup mixed berries (strawberries, blueberries, raspberries)
- 1 tablespoon chia seeds
- 1/2 cup coconut water
- 1/2 cup almond milk
- 1 teaspoon honey (optional)

Instructions:

1. Combine mixed berries, chia seeds, coconut water, almond milk, and honey in a blender.
2. Blend until the chia seed magic is achieved.
3. Pour into a glass and enjoy the antioxidant-rich delight!

Nutrition Information:

- Calories: 160

- Protein: 4g
- Carbohydrates: 34g
- Fat: 3g
- Fiber: 8g
- Sugar: 20g
- Portion Size: 1 serving

Avocado and Kale Power Smoothie

Ingredients:

- 1/2 avocado, peeled and pitted
- 1 cup kale leaves, stems removed
- 1/2 cup cucumber, sliced
- 1/2 lemon, juiced
- 1/2 cup coconut water

Instructions:

1. Combine avocado, kale, cucumber, lemon juice, and coconut water in a blender.
2. Blend until the creamy green power is achieved.
3. Pour into a glass and revel in the nourishing avocado and kale fusion!

Nutrition Information:

- Calories: 180
- Protein: 5g
- Carbohydrates: 30g
- Fat: 7g
- Fiber: 8g
- Sugar: 15g
- Portion Size: 1 serving

Watermelon Mint Cooler

Ingredients:

- 2 cups fresh watermelon, cubed
- A handful of fresh mint leaves
- 1/2 lime, juiced
- 1/2 cup coconut water
- Ice cubes (optional)

Instructions:

1. Combine watermelon, mint leaves, lime juice, coconut water, and ice cubes in a blender.
2. Blend until the refreshing watermelon mint cooler is achieved.

3. Pour into a glass and stay cool with this hydrating treat!

Nutrition Information:

- Calories: 100
- Protein: 2g
- Carbohydrates: 24g
- Fat: 1g
- Fiber: 3g
- Sugar: 18g
- Portion Size: 1 serving

CONCLUSION

As we wrap up this journey through the pages of our "Diabetic Vegan Cookbook for Type 2 Diabetes," it's not just the end of a book; it's the beginning of a healthier, more vibrant lifestyle. The recipes contained within these chapters aren't merely culinary delights; they are a roadmap to transforming your relationship with food, reshaping habits, and embracing the power of mindful, nourishing choices.

In these pages, we've embarked on a flavorful exploration, proving that managing type 2 diabetes can be both delicious and satisfying. From the vibrant colors of our breakfast bowls to the hearty goodness of our dinner recipes, each dish is a testament to the joy of plant-based eating.

The 30-day meal plan has laid a foundation for sustainable habits, guiding you through weeks of diverse, nutrient-packed meals. We've discovered the art of crafting satisfying breakfasts, wholesome lunches, and delightful dinners—all without compromising on taste. The snacks, desserts, and smoothies are not just treats; they're tools for redefining how we snack, indulge, and refresh.

But this isn't just a cookbook; it's an invitation to a lifestyle rooted in wellness. The conclusion isn't the end; it's a call to continue this culinary adventure, to explore new flavors, and to experiment with plant-based creations. Celebrate the successes, no matter how small, and use them as stepping stones to a healthier you.

As you close this book, remember that every meal is an opportunity to nourish your body and soul. Embrace the journey ahead, armed with the knowledge that your kitchen is a sanctuary for health, and your choices are the building blocks of a vibrant life. Here's to your well-being, to delicious meals, and to the continuation of a mindful, diabetic vegan lifestyle. Cheers to a future filled with health, flavor, and the joy of good food!